CYNTHIA

Also by Bernard Breakell:

Falmouth at War

CYNTHIA

The Life Story
of a Quadriplegic
Born with Cerebral Palsy

Bernard Breakell

UNITED WRITERS
Cornwall

UNITED WRITERS PUBLICATIONS LTD
Ailsa, Castle Gate, Penzance, Cornwall.

British Library Cataloguing in Publication Data
Breakell, Bernard
Cynthia: the life story of a quadriplegic
born with cerebral palsy.
I. Title
362.43092

ISBN 1 85200 036 8

Printed in Great Britain by
United Writers Publications Ltd
Cornwall

In memoriam
of Cynthia and her Mum,
by the sole survivor
of a very proud family,
Bernard Breakell.

Foreword

This is to be the story of the lifespan and life-style of my late daughter, Cynthia Breakell, who was born a quadriplegic, with a distinct trace of cerebral palsy, although as you read through the ensuing chapters you will see the diagnosis was not known at the time. Cynthia was born in 1938 and died in 1988, and so I am going to unfold fifty years of experience which will contain episodes of pain, despair and − would you believe it − many delights! The idea of this exposition is to give hope, contentment and a sense of satisfaction to those parents similarly placed to my late wife and myself.

I would like to point out that I find it impossible to relate the following chapters without referral to the parents, but would seek the understanding of readers that it is especially Cynthia that we write about, and you will eventually denote that she, Cynthia, would not have survived without Mum and Dad. It is also necessary to appreciate that fifty years ago very little was known about prenatal studies and pre-birth conditions. In fact, as this story unfolds you will see that Cynthia was born just twenty years too soon, so that she was unable to take advantage of the modern scopes which were becoming available and which are still being improved upon.

I cannot finish this foreword without mentioning the

great help and encouragement which has been offered by my four friends, Jean and Walter Trevena, and David and Nona Hillier.

Chapter One

Cynthia was born on July 3rd, 1938, in the Alexandra Maternity Home, Devonport. This was well known and considered to be the best of such suitable units available at the time. I gathered it was a long and not easy birth, but all seemed to be well and we all looked forward to getting installed into our home.

The following few weeks were a trial. Somehow we could not get Cynthia to sleep at night and despite everything we tried, it was obvious that some disorder was prevalent. However this situation did quieten down eventually, and we felt able to devote more time to Cynthia and it became very apparent at the age of six months that she was not making the usual progress one would expect. This was also noticed by my own and my wife's parents.

We had long talks about the situation and decided to approach our family doctor. He considered that Cynthia was definitely backward and if there was no improvement in three months time we should arrange to talk the matter over again; which we did, because there was little improvement in Cynthia's condition. Arising out of this I asked the doctor if he would agree to a second opinion which he readily did, and then it was my own suggestion to go to the 'top', and to a most eminent child specialist we went, in Devonshire Place,

London W1, next door to Harley Street.

By now Cynthia was almost twelve months old, and we were able to manage our appointment with the specialist quite well, but her resultant prognosis was quite devastating to us as parents. We were informed that she had suffered some brain damage at birth, that she would never walk or be able to support herself in any way. She would never be able to see properly and would need the constant help of a companion to assist her through life. Well, we had asked for the best opinion and we had to suffer it. We had decided in our chagrin to carry on and hope that something would crop up for us all. The longer this spell of inactivity went on the more determined we were that there must be some degree of compensatory relief for our girl.

I will have to digress for a moment and to reflect that, apart from the opinion given by the specialist, I had probed and probed to find out why this condition to Cynthia had happened, and I was continually put down by all the medics that there must have been difficulties at the birth which perhaps demanded more attention for the mother as opposed to the new infant. I could never break down this theory and, to be rather crude, I felt that some sort of medical cover-up was being adopted. This situation need not happen in these days and times.

Having been to London and reported back to our doctor who had received the specialist's opinion, he too felt sorry and that there was nothing more to be done. If there was any consolation at all, he felt we should try to achieve another addition to the family so that he or she could grow up to support Cynthia as she grew older. I must say, what an outlook, because at the back of our minds we felt that this was too risky an adventure, in the light of the fact that we could not establish absolute cause and effect of the present situation.

However the foregoing experience did not mean we were going to give up. My wife and I were still relatively young and energetic and we decided to wait and hope and trust for some other opportunity to arise.

Chapter Two

By now World War II was upon us, and 1940 brought another change in our lives. I was drafted from Devonport to Falmouth supposedly for six weeks but it did not work out like that, and in view of our particular concern, together with the incessant bombing of Plymouth and Devonport, I became most anxious to achieve the transfer of Cynthia and my wife to the Falmouth area. I do not wish to pursue such circumstances other than to say that eventually I was able to rent a small property in Falmouth. And now, of course, we were faced with signing up with a new doctor and explaining our family problems with him.

Our new doctor was a Dr McKeirnan who, when he heard of our problem child, immediately arranged to have us all up at the Falmouth Hospital so that the combined unit could take a look at Cynthia and help him to ascertain how best to cope with the situation. It was a completely new innovation and approach to our problem. Apart from prescribing several tablets to steady up a slight convulsive situation, it was suggested that Cynthia ought to be wearing a spinal jacket to keep her spine more straight since the actual curvature therein should be overcome to some extent. This became a problem, but not insurmountable. The doctor had contacted a firm of medical aids in Plymouth and we were off on the road again. First of all to have this jacket measured for, then, in three weeks, to have it fitted. Poor Cynthia, it was one hell of a contraption to wear and get used to. We all felt very miserable but we felt we should try. My wife had all sorts of problems in coping with the skin rubbing and irritation to Cynthia's body. In twelve months Cynthia had grown and another jacket was demanded; and so the process went on.

My sister, who lived in Manchester, had news of an osteopath who was carrying out so-called miraculous cures and adjustments to body disorders and very forcibly suggested we visit him. We talked it over and we felt we ought not to pass up any chance. But I first of all sought the advice of Dr McKeirnan, who I felt would not readily agree, and so to be fair to him I offered to visit his best recommended child specialist as well, making a round trip of it, and feeling perhaps that some new medical science may have come forward.

When all the arrangements had been made we set off for Harley Street, this time, and then proceeded to Manchester. Our visit to Harley Street gave us no compensation at all — quite disappointing. Arriving in Manchester we arranged to stay for one week and during that time we visited the osteopath on two occasions.

He certainly appeared to sustain a touch and we rather felt that Cynthia had become more erect as opposed to tending to be over to one side. Grasping at any chance of improvement I arranged for him to come down to Plymouth and we would meet him at my parents' house in Devonport, having previously travelled up from Falmouth. We did this on three occasions but the cost of it all was becoming more than we could readily absorb. Despite everybody's show of confidence in the treatment I was definitely not convinced and eventually my wife agreed with me. We had definitely been duped, the only satisfaction being that we tried. Dr McKeirnan proved to be right, and so we went on, but remained hopeful that something would turn up.

Dr McKeirnan died quite suddenly, and we were faced with registering with another doctor. We chose Dr Shier of Penryn, who became a great friend of the family, so to speak, apart from being a most attentive doctor especially as far as our daughter was concerned. The year was 1946 and Cynthia was growing bigger and heavier. She needed a new spinal jacket again and Dr Shier considered this should be carried out under the National Health. Accordingly he arranged for an orthopaedic surgeon to visit Cynthia. By arrangement we were asked to attend at the City Hospital, Truro, to have a plaster cast made for her back. I personally could not understand this, and when I posed the question I was told sharply to leave it to the surgeon. Within a month we were asked to attend the hospital again for a fitting of the new jacket. It was as I felt in the beginning, a complete misinterpretation of the intended purpose of such a medical aid. The jacket itself fitted exactly to the shape of the back and did nothing to straighten the curvature. We asked Dr Shier to call and take note of the situation. Quite simply he took the jacket off Cynthia and carried it outside to the dustbin, saying, "Well, we did try folks! so what do we do now?" and I replied, "We do nothing except give the lass six months to live in peace." He said, "I quite agree, but we must monitor the situation weekly and note what happens." But Cynthia produced a smile upon her face which we had not seen for ages. At last she felt free, and we could discern all sorts of features within her which were beginning to change to a happy nature despite her many inabilities. Had we made the right decision? I felt in my bones that we had.

Chapter Three

I think a little diversification from all the foregoing is demanded and so I shall devote this chapter to the very different side of Cynthia and one which made her an absolute angel to all who came into contact with her. Of course, there were a lot of people who did not want to know her or get interested in her. But let us forget those and I think I may well surprise you.

We shall begin by describing a typical day of her life with Mum, because obviously I had to be away running a business to provide for us. So, it was up at 8.30 to 9.00 am each day when she would be sat on the toilet and given a complete overall wash then dressed. My wife had worked out a system of so doing and at that time was quite capable of handling and lifting Cynthia. I must ask you to realise that our patient was incapable of doing anything to help herself, she had to be fed and closely helped in every possible manner. By now, between them, Cynthia and her Mum had established their language which by the way was an innovation. So that if Cynthia wished to go to the toilet, she knew what she had to signify, and by golly in this particular situation you would, I feel sure, appreciate such significance. I would further this point by recording that our girl would become most upset if there was ever an 'accident' so to speak. But this was number one aspect in all our favours, thanks to Mum's persistence. As a part of Cynthia's day and time-table she would be given toilet facilities at 8.30 am, 1.00 pm, 5.30 pm and 9.30 pm. She was trained to this and looked forward to it. But I would add that as she became older and much more sensible she also became more adjustable to specific timing. We had reached the stage where a little persuasion and chat would work wonders.

By the way, actual bathing was carried out two or three times a week and was appreciated, but it took the two of us — Mum and Dad — to carry out this operation. We had no help at all at this stage. Around the house Cynthia had the use of a push-chair or she would sit well propped up in her armchair. She was now eight to nine years old, enjoyed the radio with plays, soap operas and music, which became a self education to her. She also enjoyed the life in the kitchen with Mum and took a surprising interest into what was being prepared for meals etc. By now, I am very pleased to report that her speech had improved to the stage that a reasonable attempt to establish a brief and fairly sensible conversation could be achieved. Her hearing was faultless, and she could see things, not very well, but if you recall the days when we visited those London specialists, well, they were not quite right. Things were to improve thanks to heaven. She also began to reveal a capable memory which became better and better, much to our amazement. You will hear more about this later.

Nevertheless, with all the aforementioned little advantages, for which we were very grateful, my wife and I still realised that her inability to show any effort to crawl, walk or give any useful use of the arms and legs was definitely going to result in a trial of strength and character for all hands. Cynthia's general nature demanded all that strength and we were determined to give it all the way. At the same time we

16

were ever watchful and vigilant for any news that would help
our situation.

Chapter Four

Our next effort to try and achieve some help for Cynthia came in 1949. Into Penryn there came to reside a specialist and I happened to be carrying out some work at his residence. I mentioned my dilemma about Cynthia, and he said he would be most interested to come and see her providing it would not upset our own doctor. A word with Dr Shier and he immediately agreed and concurred. He also added that he would, of course, like to hear of the specialist's prognosis of the case.

Accordingly a visit was arranged and the specialist spent a lot of time probing, reflecting back, but in the end he could not give us any hopeful news. He did, however, suggest that we might like to take Cynthia up to Ravencourt Park, London, to the Royal Masonic Hospital, to have some tests carried out and be able to receive news of the latest facilities for such cases. We agreed to travel. The specialist said he would talk to Dr Shier and that he would make all the arrangements at the Royal Masonic for Cynthia's admittance. Apparently the specialist had some close associationship with the hospital. Within a week we were on our way. We had arranged that my wife would stay in London so that she could keep in touch with the situation.

It must be remembered that this was our 'patient's' first

time for a stay in hospital and we did not quite know what to expect. Incidentally, I had to return to Falmouth with arrangements of course to keep closely in touch. She was admitted on a Sunday afternoon and we left her feeling quite uncomfortable. I took my wife to her place of abode and then drove back to Falmouth. It perhaps should be stated that I was in a hectic state of business at that time and could not afford to neglect it.

My wife telephoned me on the following Tuesday evening to say that Cynthia was comfortable but not happy. Certain tests had been carried out and the results were awaited. On the Thursday night my wife rang to say she had had a long chat with the specialist dealing with the case and that we were not going to be able to look forward to any positive results. Also that Cynthia was very miserable, not eating or co-operating in any respect.

My decision was quick and abrupt, and I asked my wife to obtain Cynthia's release and told her that I would be with them by lunch-time on the Friday. And so it was, and we drove back to Falmouth and felt glad to be home. Once again we were glad to see a smile on our girl's face. But now came the inquest which did not have a very good aspect or outlook. To cut the situation short, it had not been a very successful innings so to speak, but once again we had tried. My wife and I felt we were coming to the end of our tether and also felt that we should be thinking to the future, but perhaps with a lot of hesitation. At this stage of the game, if you could call it such, we always felt willing to have a go, clutching at straws. My biggest frustration in all this is that we could never ever apportion the actual reason for such a disaster. Hence the remarks in my foreword; our girl was born twenty years before medical science began to sit up and take notice.

We, as a family were not quite happy, but feeling that we

must put up with things and make the best of it. My wife and I had long talks and felt we must try to make life as easy as we could for the future. At this particular time we were missing out on a lot of life's social gatherings and so forth, but we felt we had a duty to pursue and must adhere to this. Our first step towards being futuristic was to build a new bungalow with all sorts of making life easy aspects which would help our problems.

It was at this stage that Cynthia became very ill with a mysterious stomach complaint. Our doctor could not fathom the problem despite making several tests. At one period she became so ill that we thought we were going to lose her and only just in time intervention by Dr Shier and a cortisone intravenous injection saved her life. We all sat sweating it out for two hours to note if this injection was to have the desired effect, and it did. She became noticeably better but still there remained traces of the stomach disorder. I had an idea which I put to Dr Shier who, incidentally, was very frustrated and worried. Cynthia was worried too, psychologically she began to feel that she was never going to get out of the house again.

I have to digress here to tell you that as one part of our plans for the future we had bought and renovated an old cottage in Devon on the edge of Dartmoor. The idea being that we could use it for a weekend getaway. It had an acre of land, was semi-isolated and there was plenty of space to get Cynthia outside without being overlooked by some folk who could not appreciate our position. We found we had to put up with a lot of stupid behaviour by some people who had not had a problem liken to ours. Our very close friends were much more understanding than this, I hasten to add.

Now back to the original idea. This little cottage was close to the Dame Hannah Rogers Home for Spastics, near Ivybridge, and I felt they must have a consultant physician looking after their patients with all the experience of cerebral palsy. Dr Shier telephoned them and made contact with this consultant, and an appointment was made for him to come and see Cynthia at our cottage and Dr Shier most kindly offered to come as well. We had to make plans for this because Cynthia was in poor shape really to make the journey but we felt it was worth the effort. So the back of the car was filled with cushions and pillows and the girl was comfortably laid out in the back, and we made it to our destination with six days to spare before our date with the consultant which was on a Friday, with Dr Shier to travel up on the morning of that day. Those six days worked wonders. Our girl slept throughout, mostly out on a camp-bed in the garden, the weather was very kind to us and psychologically it had a desired effect. Dr Shier could not believe his eyes when he saw her. It was so good of him to travel all that way and was something we as parents would never forget. Conclusively, when the consultant arrived and he and Dr Shier got together, they went into all the aspects of the case and then took us parents to one side with all the explanations. We were not going to achieve wonderful things but the consultant had advised Dr Shier how he could perhaps overcome this stomach ailment. And so we broke up and went home to Cornwall.

Cynthia did eventually improve in health generally, then came back that old smile upon her features again. What an experience it all was.

I am afraid I took the initiative next, in saying that we should not be travelling the country again except, of course, to stay at our little cottage. I could denote signs of some strain upon my wife and the year was now around 1960. We moved into our new bungalow at Penryn and proceeded to settle down for a while, life had been so disturbing and worrying, a spell of peace was due to us. I could see more problems ahead, and the fact that I may well have to retire early. Consequently I decided that I must get working to accumulate some finances for the future. Cynthia was much better in herself and she was talking better, learning a lot from the radio both in listening to plays, etc., and especially music, oh yes. This was going to be very apparent in a few years time and I shall be devoting a chapter to this end in which I think I shall astonish some folk.

Chapter Five

So the next few years became a devotion to duty, so to speak. All work and not much play. Cynthia was holding out quite well and we had bought her a new, modern wheel-chair which appeared to give her much pleasure. And I have to say life was a bit easier for Mum and Dad as far as she was concerned. Our immediate neighbours around us began to get used to her ways and it was not long before she had imposed her presence upon them. I now feel I must introduce to you two young friends who were eventually to play a great part in Cynthia's life and were obviously helpful to Mum and Dad. They were Jean and Walter Trevena. Jean had been my secretary in business, and Walter had been our Company Secretary and Director in business. Always good friends and younger company, so to speak. To our subject they became Auntie Jean and Uncle Walter. They had a daughter named Heather and she and Cynthia became good associates. I have to say here that it was not everyone who understood Cynthia's little mannerisms and ways, but this trio certainly took an interest. They will again be referred to much later in this book and especially as our general needs became greater.

Our knowledge and memory box (Cynthia), as I used to call her, always had something new to tell me when I arrived home and never ceased to amaze me. Being a busy man it was sometimes late at night when all was quiet for the day, and I could sit and think that if she had only been normal we would have a brilliant subject upon us. My wife and I tried very hard to consider how we could emulate on her brilliance but the fact that she could not walk or have the use of her hands and arms made the situation impossible, because those very facts meant that she always had to have someone at her side. For instance, if she wanted to blow her nose or she had an itchy ear, or the sleeves of her cardigan had slipped below the normal wearing height, then it became action stations. One of the worst things that could happen to us was for Cynthia to catch a nasal cold. This would be a full time attendance job.

Time was moving on and it was 1967-68. I could now note positive signs of a breakdown in my wife's health and, having regard to all things, I thought it would be wise to move back into Devon and somewhere near where my wife's relatives lived. Accordingly, after deep discussion, we applied for permission to build a bungalow upon the one acre site of our existing cottage. This eventually became approved and within two years we had built the bungalow to a standard that we considered would suit all our needs for the rest of our lives.

I was now considering semi-retirement, Cynthia was keeping reasonably well, and for Mum, I hoped, the new environment would help her, with me more able to assist her.

We carried out the move which went faultlessly. Having settled in nicely, we were faced with registering with a new doctor: not so easy. I suppose we telephoned up to four doctors who did not want to know when we mentioned that an invalid child was involved. The excuse offered was that if a night call was requested, they would find it difficult to respond. Even this same response came from the doctor in the village. This, I am afraid, shook our faith in human nature, besides the fact that we felt terribly alone and isolated. Actually, if it had not been for my wife's influence I would have exposed these circumstances to the local press.

My wife had a brilliant idea and contacted the Dame Hannah Rogers Home and asked if they could recommend a suitable physician. Once again they came across with the right sort of doctor and I made the contact, we had our interview and he said he would be along to see Cynthia as soon as he had time, and of course Mum and Dad became part of the whole new registration.

The doctor came to see Cynthia and immediately recommended that we sought the use of an invalid hoist. Actually I had had the foresight to prepare for the use of such equipment in the design of the bungalow. He organised for us to visit two hospitals where the use of such hoists were in action, and of course we had to try to conform. You see, he, the doctor, was concerned that the lifting of the patient was becoming detrimental to our own systems. It became a very wise move. We should have been able to achieve such equipment on the National Health Service but I feared, upon enquiries, that Mum and Dad would be long gone into hospital with hernias before a hoist was given to us. All right, so once again we must fend for ourselves. We were quite used to this by now and a few telephone calls established the type of hoist most suitable for us at Torquay. We drove up there and brought it back with us together with all the requisite equipment. Very soon we had it in operation and Cynthia was quite elated with the outcome. I must say that I first of all accepted it as a bore because of the extra time it took to move Cynthia around, but I knew in my heart of hearts we were going to have to submit to this and look to the future.

Life was beginning to take on a new look for us, and in the

b

light of the fact that lifting our patient around was supposedly to become extinct I had to consider the purchase
of a suitable car, which with alterations, would accommodate
Cynthia and also keep my wife driving in comfort. It took
some time, thought and minor engineering, and we finished
up with an adapted Citreon Safari Estate. Let us not dwell
upon this, because the cost made me feel very low and a little
bit disgruntled. But it was all very necessary to our survival
as a family.

Now I ask, having regard to similarly placed families, what
can one do to help oneself without the wherewithal — cash?
There is definitely insufficient funds from the National
Health Service forthcoming in these very essential cases.
Perhaps the circumstances are a little better now, in the days
twenty years on. I consider my efforts and outcries as being
pioneering.

Chapter Six

Having become settled in our Devonshire home we had expected to have some support to our cause from my wife's sister and family. This did not appear to be forthcoming, so I shall not refer to it again. However, readers of this story may well be wondering what plans we had arranged for Cynthia in the event of my wife or I becoming inactive, so to speak. After all, we were both approaching the age of sixty and had been living under great strain.

So once again we thought and considered hard and long and finished up arranging to go back to Falmouth to stay with Jean and Walter for a few days. As a result of this we were able to arrange a meeting with my late partners in business and their wives. They all knew Cynthia very well and especially so as far as Jean and Walter Trevena were concerned. The other two were David Hillier and his wife Nona. They knew Cynthia quite well, but having a relatively young family at the time could never really give sufficient support to our girl. However, we laid before them our thoughts and asked if they felt they could act as trustees for Cynthia's welfare in the event of any possible breakdown as far as we — Mum and Dad — were concerned. They all responded magnificently and my wife and I felt relieved and went back to Devon again. I made this quite legal by an insertion in both our wills which would also take care of any finances needed for Cynthia's welfare. The whole arrangement was the best we could do at the time. It would be reviewed, we all said, in the event of any change in circumstances.

We were able to settle down now and we made a few new friends, with Jean and Walter coming up at least every four to five weeks. David and Nona would call if in the district. And then came a calamity when my wife fell ill, finishing up with an operation in hospital and me summoned to see the surgeon. Before I saw him I had seen my wife and she was very upset about something. However, I saw the surgeon and he told me that during the course of the operation he had detected a cervical growth which proved to be cancerous and inoperable. He said he had asked a colleague, who was a radiotherapist, to see my wife. I asked him if he had told my wife of his findings and he said, "No, that is up to you now." I had to make my mind up quickly on my way back to the ward and in view of her very upset state I decided not to be ruthless. I also saw the radiotherapist and he said he would have to see my wife for treatment daily, and that I could take her home for the time being. Of course, I was shaken up too, but eventually I was able to quieten down the situation. Cynthia was extremely good, she knew something was extraordinarily wrong and used her utmost tact not to ask too many questions. When we had settled Mum down and I was getting Cynthia into bed I had a quiet chat with her and told her she was going to be busy taking Mum to hospital daily to help make her better. This consoled her, she had reached the stage where she did not like being left out of the scene. And so, as far as I was concerned, 'Blessed are the Peace-makers', but I assure you I felt far from happy. I decided that my job was to be a morale booster for the time being.

Apart from all our problems, this book is about Cynthia and her behaviour and reactions to certain crises, and I have to say that she was marvellous and the least possible trouble, it was as if she knew that she ought to co-operate.

The following few months were not without problems but my wife certainly progressed to the state where she could live a pretty reasonable life. However, this radiotherapy treatment had taken toll of some of her normal functions and it became something we all had to live with. Once again I have to say that we had less problems with Cynthia than for many years, but I found that I was gradually taking over her care and maintenance.

So, to progress with time, a few years passed on until the next crisis, when my wife had to go into hospital again for some early treatment after which she was given an extended period of life, up until a major operation became necessary. I regret I have to at least briefly refer to these circumstances but shortly you will note how it affected our main subject. Cynthia obviously had grown older whilst all these problems were going on and by this I mean she had collected in her little brain experiences which if I could have avoided I would have.

In 1982 our family became sadly disorganised by my wife's illness and by November of that year I was beginning to think we were fighting a losing battle. Jean came up to visit us for a day and pretty soon summed up the situation that I too was beginning to wilt a little bit. She decided, with the co-operation of her husband Walter, that she should stay with us for a while and so she took over my wife's care and I devoted all my time to Cynthia, who I must say had been a little neglected without the least complaint from her.

My wife unfortunately passed away in early December 1982. We were able to isolate Cynthia from the last few days, but she knew, she knew! I was now faced with telling her what had happened to her Mum, of course, in the most tactful way, and she was a little brick, very few tears, and I

29

said she would now have to take over the role of looking after Dad. I would have preferred to have seen a few more tears really, but they were not forthcoming. She now had a job to do and she became hell bent on doing it. There were other things on my mind which had to be kept to myself until after the funeral. As regards the funeral, it was not possible to include Cynthia in these arrangements for service at church. We arranged for her to stay at home in the care of a friend and they prepared a simple meal for the return of the mourners. This kept her occupied.

The next couple of days were a bit upsetting. Jean of course had to be getting back to her home in Falmouth and I was faced with a dilemma as to whether Cynthia and I would have to part company. For instance, would she be better off and cared for in a suitable Home or could I manage to keep us together. It did not take long for me to reach a decision and I decided that providing the local service officials accepted my proposals, I was going to make a damned good effort to look after Cynthia. After all, I had been virtually doing it for the last two years and placing her in a Home would have been a heartbreaker for both of us. I enlisted the support of our doctor who felt I was doing the correct thing providing I could keep fit and well enough. He arranged for us to have the services of a nurse to help me with the bathing once a week. She would also keep a vigilant eye on Cynthia and myself. I was also able to arrange for the services of a lady from the nearby village to come up and keep the bungalow clean and tidy. This was to be our new way of life. I have to say that I knew Cynthia was missing her Mum but she never murmured. Jean and Walter came pretty regularly once a month to visit us and check upon any needs.

Before proceeding further with this story, I would like to relate the following as something which will remain everlastingly in my memory. Jean and I knew that Cynthia was disappointed at not being able to take part in Mum's funeral service and then she (Jean) came up with a wonderful idea which I quite concurred with. It was to hold a 'Strewing' ceremony of my late wife's ashes over the orchard part of our garden. I talked to Cynthia about this and it seemed to sort of appease the situation. So it was all arranged for one Sunday afternoon. Jean and Walter, Nona and David (Cynthia's four trustees) came up from Falmouth and there was myself, Cynthia and the local vicar who was to officiate over a miniature funeral service. He got well started until he was interrupted by our girl with expressions like "Ashes to ashes, dust to dust", "Our Father which art in Heaven" and "The Blessing of God Almighty". He stopped, turned to Cynthia and said "Do you want me to go through the whole of the Service Cynthia?" and she said, "Yes, please," and remained silent until Amen at the end. Well, I am nearly ashamed to say that we all felt like having a little giggle, but it proved to all of us present that she had a very determined mind and once again showed evidence of her memory. She always listened intently to any relayed services on television. I was very proud of her incidentally. This action satisfied her and I am certain it gave her a sense of responsibility in that she had done her bit. I perhaps ought to say that Jean was in business in her own right as a very qualified Funeral Director.

31

Chapter Seven

I must move on now and perhaps explain how we were going to manage our lives. For it was a full time effort looking after Cynthia and so I had to enlist some help with our very large garden. I also had to consider that our form of transport was becoming a bit difficult for me. You will understand, I am sure, that in order to keep my girl at home I had at all times to try and remain fit. So in conference with Jean and Walter on one of their visits we arranged to buy a new Renault van, and to have it altered suitably to comply with our needs. In fact they borrowed a similar vehicle and brought it up to Devon for me to survey and make sure we were on the right track. I gave them 'carte-blanche' to proceed and within a few weeks they delivered to me this improvised vehicle with accessories, which was going to make my life easier and in turn Cynthia's. Just one thing to complete a successful exercise; I had to purchase a new car transit wheel-chair. So now Cynthia had her own transport fleet. A wheel-chair for around the house and a wheel-chair for the new van which did not have swivel wheels in the front. It is difficult to progress with this explanation but it was a very necessary acquisition to our survival. Thank God for Jean and Walter, they had done us proud.

Not without thought at times of the loss of our Mum

we ploughed on. We had to work out ways of managing our weekly shopping and we shopped at establishments where I could always be in sight of Cynthia, who had now become used to staying in the new van. She was never left in it for more than ten minutes at a time and she co-operated fully. She knew that she also had a part to play. We felt a bit short of company at times but we were not made of the material to feel sorry for ourselves. For the next three years we managed quite well.

We had a good sequence of nurses and a good health visitor, and an excellent doctor. About twice a year we would venture down to Falmouth and stay with Jean and Walter for a few days, which made a nice change and they gave me just a little relief from the situation. Cynthia would look forward to getting out and about with Jean on her own. Glad in her small way to be rid of the old fellow! When we were staying down there Jean would lay on some musical evenings of varied music but which I am pleased to say did not overawe our girl, in fact she was able to surprise us after hearing the first two or three bars of any piece. We were all in agreement that it was quite an amazing sequence and it appeared to give Cynthia immense pleasure and all of us too. I hope you will remember a significant programme on television, it was called 'Name That Tune', in which contestants were given the opportunity to name certain tunes played by the orchestra, and in which if you could put correct names to three tunes you would win a car. Our Cynthia became a great competitor and she would have won five cars out of six efforts. It was amazing, I would sit and watch the expression upon her face, and very frankly I have to say that I did not know the answers, but I knew by that facial expression that she knew that she was coming out with the correct answer. If the tune being played extended over five to six bars I knew she was floundering − in the light of what I have written beforehand you will note this situation only happened once out of six times. There was nothing I could do to air this situation, it was just a phenomenon to be enjoyed by ourselves.

Once again I have to refer to this brilliant exposition of talent, music and memory-wise. It never failed to give pleasure to all our friends who were amazed and somewhat mystified. There is little doubt in anybody's mind that if Cynthia had not been handicapped in the way she was, she would have been scheduled for exceptional treatment.

Life went on, it was not always filled with rapturous occurrences but all of a sudden I contracted a bad dose of influenza through which I had to fight to keep going, and I felt extremely worried for fear that Cynthia would become involved. With the help of our doctor we came out on top. There was another occasion also when we were staying with Jean in Falmouth that I became ill with such a bug and this time it did transfer to Cynthia. Thanks to Jean, who was also thankful that we were staying with her and not in Devon, and thanks to the doctor in Falmouth, who gave us prompt attention in the light of the fact that we were visitors to the town, we pulled through again.

We floundered on for a few weeks having arrived back in Devon and then one evening disaster struck again. I was preparing Cynthia for bed at about 10 pm, brought forward our hoist to lift her to the toilet when the pump lever became detached from the main post − a weld had broken down. I made the girl comfortable and then sat to consider what best to do − 10 pm is not the best of times to achieve some help. I had an idea and rang the police, spoke to the sergeant and explained my predicament − "Well how do you think we can help?" he said. I said, "If you could allow two of your constables to come out here as soon as possible, lift by hand and strength my daughter on to her toilet and then on to her bed I shall be forever thankful, I will talk to them and sort of instruct and encourage." "We shall be with you shortly," was the reply. And so it came to pass, in ten minutes the doorbell was ringing and we had the help of two very fine policemen. Cynthia had sat quietly listening to all the telephone talk and this was going to be a new experience for her, she was fine. The constables soon had her conveyed on to the toilet and then on to her bed and well tucked in. She thanked them no end and they were delighted, they had a cup of tea and then went back on duty, saying they would call again when in the district. They had fallen in love with our girl and she had made friends for life.

Oh well, that was a good move, but I now had to consider what was going to happen the following morning in order to get Cynthia up and dressed. I knew where I had to contact and I set out to get to work on this by 9 am. The next two hours were an experience I regret to describe.

There was an occupational therapist based at Plymouth, not far from where we lived. She was responsible for such machinery and aids which are required by people like Cynthia. I rang her at 9 am and was informed that she would not be available until 9.45 am. I explained to the receptionist that I had a problem and needed her assistance quite early. She promised to ring back as soon as the OT came in. In the meantime our girl was in trouble, she was desperate to go to the toilet and she had become quite out of routine. I talked and explained to her that we had a problem and not to worry. I padded her up and gave as much protection as I could, but Cynthia was most sensitive to such conditions.

To cut a long story short, the bed became wetted as anticipated and Cynthia was very, very upset. At 10 am our OT rang and I explained our difficulties and how urgent it had become for some positive action. She said as casually as you like, "OK, I doubt if I can do anything about another hoist until late in the afternoon." By this time, and I think for the first time in my life, I blew my top in no uncertain manner. I do not think it would be correct to steer you through an unpleasant conversation. Suffice it to say that our OT with an assistant arrived with another hoist at 11.30 am. We soon had Cynthia up, cleaned and dressed. Actually it is fair to remark that the OT did not know of the difficulties and intricacies of our manner of survival. But she certainly now knew and should have been very much more aware. After all, Cynthia was a patient of hers. I told her I should be in touch with the Health Authority to explain my experiences and the fact that they should arrange for some emergency cover for out-of-office hours. Within a fortnight I was given a number to telephone in exceptional circumstances.

This experience was nothing short of an abomination and proves the point that we are part of a special breed. If one does not play absolute 'Hell' in such circumstances one can become very down-hearted. Ultimately though, we did achieve an improvement in the service.

Within a few days, and during one of my positive thought excursions, I began to realise that it was perhaps unfair of me towards Cynthia's well-being to try to carry on as we were going. I telephoned Jean and asked if she would approve and feel better if we decided to move back to Falmouth. She was delighted because we would be under her watchful eye and said she and Walter would come up to see us as soon as possible to discuss such a move. In the meantime I placed our property in agents' hands to get the feel of the market. We very soon were receiving requests to view.

Chapter Eight

Jean and Walter visited us the following weekend and the move to Falmouth became more definite. We had to find a suitable bungalow in that area however, and by chance we both hit upon a possibility. I have previously mentioned Nona and David, the other two trustees for Cynthia. They were in possession of such a bungalow which they had been letting to visitors.

We arranged to visit Falmouth and stay at Jean's for a few days whilst we viewed this bungalow. We considered we would have to carry out certain works in order to comply with Cynthia's requirements, such as a new bathroom, new front entrance doors to accept passage of her wheel-chairs and a few more incidentals. I was now ready to make a sound and reasonable offer which was accepted forthwith providing I could dispose of our Devon home. This did not take long and I very soon received my asking price. Meantime my firm of builders were to seek planning permission for the proposed additions and alterations.

Cynthia and I had returned to Devon and immediately we began to pack up and also do the inevitable clearing out. Jean had volunteered to arrange for removal transport. We had organised to make our move to Falmouth very early in June 1986. We spent our last few days in Devon saying good-bye to our few friends and to our professional helpers such as our doctor and his team of nurses. I did not leave without some regrets and Cynthia also I believe, but for her it was to be a new life coming up. She loved being with Jean and Walter.

On the morning of our leaving, Jean and Walter had driven up from Falmouth and arrived at 9 am with the removal vans. We were on our way to Falmouth by 11.30 am. Cynthia was in her own transport driven by Walter and I was with Jean in her car. This turned out to be a very well organised exit and we were to stay at Jean and Walter's residence for two or three days whilst we achieved some new order to our new bungalow. Dare I say it, this turned out to be most disappointing. Suffice it to say we had to stay with Jean for eleven days and no further comments will be administered except for the worry of it all. Jean and Walter had to spend several evenings clearing out rubbish and cleaning up, I could not really help because I had to stay with Cynthia. However, we moved in about the middle of June and within a few days we were getting used to a new routine, though not without some problems.

I had to leave Cynthia's hoist in Plymouth for I had turned it over to the Health Authority to save me the cost of having it regularly serviced. Consequently the Cornwall Health Authority had to supply us with a new hoist, which they did. But it was not of the same type that we had been used to and quite unsuitable for use in a house situation. I complained bitterly to the department responsible but they said they could do nothing to help. What a ridiculous situation. I could see myself in hospital within a week by struggling with this awful contraption. Jean was helping us no end because she understood our difficulties. In conference, we decided to try to purchase a suitable type of hoist and within a few telephone calls we had hit upon the correct source, but we had to place the order with the firm's agents who fortunately were established in Falmouth. Within a few days we were out of trouble but I had to pay for this new machine myself to the tune of £700. I determined to write to the Health Authority and explain the complete misunderstanding of their department over our case. After all, I was saving the Authority at least £250 a week by keeping Cynthia at her own home. I demanded in the nicest possible way that they refund my outgoings in this matter. There were a few quibbles and dissensions and I had to threaten to expose the circumstances publicly. They eventually had to alter their rules a little to allow this payment to be made. Quite frankly I began to wonder whether life was worth living. However, I soon shook that feeling off.

You will be wondering how all this disruption was affecting our prime subject. We all took great care to protect her from any upsets. Jean would be taking her for outings, visiting her friends who also became friends of Cynthia. I was amazed when she would tell me after her trips who she had met, and I knew that she would never forget them, such was the state of her memory — just like a computer. All this change was good for her (and for me too, secretly), and without being unloving she was pleased to get away from me. Above all it increased her remote independence and gave her confidence.

Now comes the day when Jean had organised to take her to the final rehearsal of her favourite musical — *Oklahoma*. Jean had set her mind to take Cynthia and there was no hedging. I am going to be honest and say I would have been very reluctant to do this, but they were both full of confidence and determination. Jean had organised some help out at the Falmouth Pavilion for loading and unloading the girl, and looking at her before they set off I thought this is going to be something momentous in both their lives, and so it turned out to be. I kept busy organising a meal for when they arrived home and keeping my fingers crossed for success. I don't think either of them will regret that day — Jean for achievement and Cynthia for something she never expected to happen.

I had hoped not to have related the following but I consider it worth a mention. I had been experiencing trouble with my eyes and cataracts had been diagnosed, especially to my right eye. I felt I must organise to have some expert opinion upon this and accordingly before I left Devon I had written to the eye consultant at Falmouth asking for an appointment pretty soon after our arrival. It was all arranged but I had been worried and concerned about what would happen to Cynthia. Accordingly, during my consultation with the eye surgeon, I asked if he could arrange for a private room with accommodation for my daughter and, of course, myself. I would ask you to appreciate that this would be only the second time in her life that I would be away from her. I knew this would only be a time lapse of three to four days and that I would have the complete support of Jean and Walter who fortunately lived directly opposite the Falmouth Hospital. On the day designated for my attendance we occupied our room complete with all our equipment and anticipated any assistance we needed with Cynthia would be forthcoming from the nurses. However, Jean came up to the hospital at night to put Cynthia to bed and arrived early in the morning to get her up and dressed, and helped during the day with toilet arrangements. The nurses kept promising to come and help but, of course, were so busy it was a devastation to say the least. My operation was accomplished and we all looked forward to the signal to go home. In the end Cynthia rebelled in her own way and I knew it was time to withdraw. I shall be eternally thankful to Jean and Walter for their help in that sort of embarrassing situation.

After a few weeks of living back in Falmouth I felt I should have some help around the house generally and to do the ironing in particular — a job which I hated. Jean had noticed a shop window advert offering domestic help. I rang the telephone number and one way and another the lady in question arrived on our doorstep. I was a bit apprehensive as to whether or not she would be happy with Cynthia but she said she would give it a go. I need not have worried too much because Cynthia paved her own way into the lady's well-being; and so we have the arrival of Wendy Dean. It was not long before we knew the whole of her history, how many in her family, who her husband worked for, etc. Cynthia and her became very staunch friends and allies, both looking forward to the two mornings when they could get together. Wendy's husband Colin and her son Steven were introduced to us and it soon dawned upon me that we had new friends. Our nearby neighbours across the road introduced themselves, Jan and Rob Mullett and in no time Cynthia had additional allies. They had two sons, too, who were never afraid to speak to her. There were a few immediate neighbours however who seemed to be afraid of crossing our domain and we knew why — we had experienced it all before.

After being in residence here for about six months and having regard to our relative positions, I had become a bit futuristic. After all I was now seventy-five years of age and Cynthia forty-eight years. I felt we were not having the same support from the Health Authority that we had in Devon and so I complained of this with the result that we received a visit from a social worker. I explained that I thought that we should be receiving regular visits from a health visitor and from an occupational therapist and also from officers liken to herself. So be it, she said, and turned on the whole works so that before I knew it I felt that I too was being surveyed and rightly so I suppose, in the light of my age. I received a letter from her saying she had convened a meeting to be held at our home with all the requisite persons who should be concerned with our particular circumstances.

I told Cynthia that she was going to receive quite a few visitors and that she would be able to sit in and listen only; the following will make you smile and perhaps laugh. A doctor arrived first for a preliminary look at Cynthia and then followed the social worker, a nursing sister and a health visitor, who headed a nearby Day Centre. Jean Trevena was there as our main support and Wendy Dean, our home helper, as our second support. The meeting commenced by the introduction of names and capacities such as "I am Samantha O'Connell, Social Worker" or "I am Dr Swithen, Senior Consultant" and so forth from around the table and finishing with myself — "I am Bernard Breakell, seeking your help and advice." And then whilst everyone was clearing their throats, a little voice came out with, "I am Cynthia Breakell," which immediately invoked a titter all around. My girl was not going to be left out and by the facial countenances she had made her mark. Incidentally, as a result of this meeting I was taken to one side by the senior consultant who pledged to me that he would gladly come to visit us at any time Cynthia demanded some attention. I thought that was a wonderful gesture.

Chapter Nine

The result of the meeting, I believed, was that they were satisfied that I was still quite capable of standing by Cynthia, especially with the consistent help we were receiving from Jean, backed up by Wendy and the nurses. It was considered necessary for Cynthia to have a 'special friend' to visit her weekly, someone she could talk to and become reliant upon, to tell any troubles to and also to express any special interests which came to hand. Our Jean again came to the rescue with such a person, a Mrs Gilly Peters, who fervently took interest and who visited us once weekly when I would slip quietly out of the room and let them get interested in each other.

The next considered option was for Cynthia to visit and take part in some sessions at the Day Centre. I must admit that I was somewhat apprehensive about this but I felt I ought to co-operate. Notwithstanding my reluctance, I arranged to visit this establishment to view the atmosphere, the type of persons attending and the possibilities of loading and unloading Cynthia from and to our vehicle. I had the feeling that I must try to get our girl interested and despite another chore for me we made it on three occasions and I left her on her own or at least with some of the other patients. I have to say that I was not at all happy with the situation. Cynthia needed constant stand-by attention and she was not receiving such, despite the organiser's assurance that she had a retired nurse coming especially to give such support. Furthermore, I did not think the type of patient or inmate of this Centre was going to improve my girl's present standard of intelligence.

Now I do not remark upon this from any derogative angle. The organiser was obviously carrying out a great job with her patients but it was not going to improve Cynthia's well-being or intelligence. I had carried out the wishes of the aforesaid meeting and I would have carried on supporting the well meaning of the attendance at the centre, but all I can say is that I felt absolutely correct in my decision to withdraw. Were I pressed for reasons I would have been most discreet because this particular Centre supported by Mencap carries out a very worthwhile job.

In the meantime, our neighbours and friends had got together to lighten the load, so to speak. Jan and Rob Mullett, our neighbours directly opposite us and before mentioned, offered to take Cynthia out in her vehicle every Sunday without fail. Colin (Wendy Dean's husband) offered to take Cynthia out for a run every Monday morning. In so applying this very special application they all three realised that they would not be allowed to let the side down, so to speak. They never did either and the recipient looked forward very much to those weekly occasions. So did I. We had another gentleman in the name of David Hillier who would take her sometimes on a Saturday morning but this was never very permanent, probably because of his uncertain commitments. Cynthia sometimes found this difficult to understand but that is life and she had to appreciate it. I have spent hours trying to quell little upsets of this nature. However, by and large it worked out very well, both in relationships and the fact that she could look forward to those permanent outings. I am certain that Jan, Rob and Colin looked forward to and enjoyed the experience. Cynthia was so appreciative of such attention and she also kept them quite amused in her inimitable manner.

You will no doubt note by now that we had built up quite a nice few loyal and trusted friends and they were all good friends of each other. At times I was able to take a change and go out for a few hours. There was always someone who would sit in with Cynthia especially Jean's daughter, Heather.

Chapter Ten

We went along with this procedure for quite some time, in fact into May 1988 when Cynthia became quite ill and one Sunday afternoon I had to ask Jean to come over, which she quickly did, and we decided we ought to ask a doctor to call. Now I must explain that Cynthia always contracted a measure of phlegm, caused generally by her inability to be actually active. I was used and able to move this congestion generally first thing in the morning, but this bout of phlegm sickness persisted for about two hours during early afternoon and when the doctor arrived she was in a pretty low state. He became alarmed and insisted that she should go into hospital. Jean and I set off with her in her own transport and by the time we arrived at the hospital in Truro the sickness had stopped but she was very low and we soon had some attention, but the doctors were really at a loss to understand the cause of the upset. They insisted she was X-rayed chestwise and then they said that they could not form an opinion and that we could take her home since she had now settled down and her colour looked healthier. We were to return to the hospital if there was any recurrence.

We arrived home and we soon had her feeling comfortable and after toilet into bed. Regretfully, but most significantly, I have to relate that our visit to the hospital did nothing to enhance a re-visit. For instance, Cynthia, in accordance with her routine, wished to go to the toilet. We achieved a commode but no hoist to lift her on to it. They did not have a clue how to deal with the situation. In the end I said to the doctors and nurses, "For God's sake do what you want to do quickly with her and allow me to get home where we have all the facilities." This was rather an outburst on my behalf but I ask you and any other concerned parent to take note. The year was 1988!

The following day Jean and I decided that we should have our own doctor to come to see her. I should explain that the Sunday doctor was a locum. Our own doctor came to see us and after explaining the events of the previous afternoon said he would like a consultant chest specialist to see her and he would arrange it. He also suggested that we sought the help and advice of a physiotherapist to show us the resources which would help remove the phlegm each day. Jean knew a connection and by the evening we had a married couple on our doorstep. They were both physiotherapists and in no time Cynthia was being delightfully rolled and rolled over and well thumped in the correct places. I am pleased to say that our patient accepted the treatment and I felt able to continue the practice in the right and proper way. By the way, Cynthia had made two more friends.

The doctor was in touch with the news that a chest consultant would be calling early on the Friday morning. The consultant arrived and thoroughly examined Cynthia, but he had to admit that in this particular case and having regard to the patient's physical disadvantages, he would find it difficult to recommend any special treatment and what we were practising at the moment would be within his advice. He did, however, suggest that he would arrange to loan us a special suction machine with reservoir which when switched on electrically, would help remove the phlegm via a fine tube inserted in the throat, without asking the patient to urge too violently. Within two or three days this machine was delivered and we soon had it set up and working. It was a good appliance and Cynthia was not in the least perturbed with its use.

Cynthia's condition eventually decidedly improved and although we had a few more duties to perform nobody was grumbling and we were much appreciative of all the help and advice we had received.

Now with a few weeks of less anxiety we were approaching Cynthia's 50th birthday and all being well I was determined to make it a memorable day for her. She was a great one for entering into special occasions. Accordingly I arranged to take her out for a birthday lunch to which I had invited all her friends, associates and those connected with her well-being.

I should say that we had previously taken her out for lunch or a snack, arranged with the help and approval of the landlord at the local hostelry. So we went forth on this particular day of July 3rd determined to make it a day of days for her. Well, everyone including Cynthia enjoyed it immensely. I felt so very proud of her and her behaviour. We had scored a winning point there. So be it.

Life proceeded as normal for a few weeks and whilst the situation is normal I would like to explain that one of my specific worries was whatever would happen to Cynthia in the event of my breaking down in health or whatever. Her trustees at this time were also concerned and in such circumstances that I have mentioned would have been faced with finding a suitable Home for her. But news had been appearing that special home circumstances outside the institutions were now being assessed and provided in certain suitable areas for disabled persons to live privately. By devious but honest means I probed this situation with the

48

Social Services Department which resulted in another meeting, this time with the policymakers. They seemed quite taken with the idea providing they could also install at least another suitable disabled person and of course with chosen attendants. I would have to sell our bungalow to the Council but with the guarantee that Cynthia would remain in her own domain and would still receive the usual visitations from the people who had been looking after her such as Jean, Walter, Wendy, Colin and the rest of her friends. I think this scheme would have eventually come to fruition which would have eased the load of worry from the trustees. However, it so turned out that it was not to be.

Before moving on to what proved to be a grim experience, I think perhaps it may be of some interest to describe how we managed to take some brief holidays. In the earlier days I was only able to take a week off and in the light of Cynthia's condition we did not feel like indulging in holiday camps or hotels, so we drove up to Manchester each year for several years to stay with my sister. We could get about daily to various resorts such as Southport, Blackpool, into Yorkshire and Derbyshire. Cynthia used to enjoy this and her memory began to build up a whole new set of circumstances. You will, I hope, realise that my wife and I could both handle and carry Cynthia at this stage.

Come the time when Cynthia had outgrown this and an invalid chair became necessary, regretfully we had to terminate our visits to the north. We just found it too difficult to negotiate entry into my sister's residence and to cope there. We were, however, able to travel to my wife's relatives in Devon at some weekends, and they offered to look after Cynthia for a few days whilst we slipped away for a short break. At first we felt most apprehensive about this, but decided in the end to accept the offer on the basis that we felt Cynthia would come to no harm for three to four

49

days. We felt it would do her confidence some good, but I did not really know how we should feel. However, we did feel assured that Rene's relatives basically knew the manner in which Cynthia had been trained, so off we went to Worcestershire and we stayed for three nights. We had arranged to meet Cynthia with her Aunt and Uncle near Exeter on our return journey. All worked out according to plan and we were glad to arrive back though obviously thankful for the break. Cynthia was not in the best of clean order when we returned, Aunt and Uncle had done their best but the handling proved more difficult than they had anticipated. Consequently Rene and I decided that that was the end of that, and forever after we would stay together.

There was an occasion later on when I applied to Social Services enquiring of their holiday home schemes and Cynthia was offered a fortnight at a county home at Yelverton. Before committing ourselves we paid a visit, and I can quickly relate that this Centre was definitely unsuitable for a person of Cynthia's stature and inability to carry out her personal needs by herself.

In the summer of 1978 and feeling the need for a change, we followed up upon a newspaper advert which described a bungalow on a farm near Hereford. My wife had two telephone conversations explaining our problems and the owners of the property fairly convinced us that we would be able to manage easy access and it all sounded very nice. Actually it turned out to be a fairly new bungalow, furnished with second-hand furniture including beds, etc. However, we spent a couple of days travelling around the area, and we were not managing Cynthia's equipment too easily. On the third day, after a pretty restless and uncomfortable night, we decided to pack and travel back home feeling pretty fed up. We left without any fuss and blaming ourselves for being too anxious for a break.

This brings me to a conclusive point that there ought to be more facilities and accommodation available throughout the country for disabled people and their carers. I do believe that in the last few years there has been an increase in interest in this area.

So life went on, and we made the best of a day as it presented itself. When we moved to the Plymouth area we were able, perhaps twice a year, to travel down to Falmouth and stay with Jean and Walter. They both went to all sorts of trouble to make life easier for us all. Later, my wife Rene's illness eliminated any thoughts of holidays for quite some time to come. After a while, during Rene's better spells, we were able to slip down to Falmouth and we would be looked after and rather spoilt.

Chapter Eleven

It was now early August 1988 and Cynthia became rather congested once again. The new machine we had at hand was very useful in clearing the phlegm situation. I called the doctor to her again and he suggested a course of antibiotics which really appeared to do no good. After a few days I felt the doctor should see her again and he did, and prescribed more antibiotics and added that he felt he could not do anything more. Actually we were getting Cynthia up and sat her upright in her armchair to help with her breathing as you would with anyone with a bronchial complaint. Right at this stage I did not feel too worried, because having had so many anxious times with her I knew she would be fighting back. But this situation persisted and it became a night and day attendance problem. This did not concern me really, I had been through it all before. I had admirable help from Jean and Wendy etc., who gave me a spell off at midday to just relieve the tension a little. The doctor came to check upon us on Friday the 12 August and said he would be away over the weekend but would ask his partner to call upon us over that time which he very attentively did.

On Sunday 14th August we were all becoming very concerned for Cynthia, I especially could not sense that fight-back spirit. Jean and Walter had a little social event on this day and by arrangement Wendy and Colin came to stand by us. After lunch I thought I should get Cynthia to the toilet and had decided to allow her to rest upon her bed for a change; she was now obviously quite poorly. On transferring her from toilet to bed by her hoist she suddenly collapsed. I asked Colin to telephone for Jean and the doctor, whilst making her comfortable on her bed, but I now feared the worst. Jean arrived, the doctor arrived, there was nothing they could do. We all of us felt so helpless. It was now 2.00 pm and our girl slipped peacefully into a coma. She passed on at 4.40 pm as always without fuss and with that inimitable smile upon her face. She at least was contented, I felt, gone off to be with her Mum.

I have to say that after fifty years of looking after her, I felt shattered but with my head upheld I survived all that self pity and felt very proud of the way we had been able to survive even after her Mum's death.

I shall be eternally grateful to friends, doctors and those who fought so wonderfully to keep Cynthia alive. There should be some medals and appreciation here because they were not dealing with a normal case. But I am sure that they are not looking for recognition, however, on their behalf I wish I had the power to grant it.

The doctors were both in agreement that Cynthia had passed on with a bronchial pneumonia which this time she had been unable to withstand. Jean proceeded to make all the funeral arrangements, but I felt with her great feeling and associationship with our girl it would be difficult for her. To this end a family friend officiated at the actual service and Jean kept my end up. At Cynthia's committal we played one of her favourite tunes, *You'll Never Walk Alone*, and she never did.

All I can say now is thanks to all the people who helped me and to those who sent wonderful letters of condolence.

I felt so very proud that Cynthia was held in such high esteem because, as I have said before, she was avoided by some due to the nature of her condition. Such is the world made up of a mixture of good doers and those who haven't got the spirit to act at all, turning their backs on adversity.

I began to settle down and review the situation after a few weeks and I concluded, in the light of what I had previously written concerning Cynthia's future should anything have happened to me, that perhaps the 'writing was on the wall' and now I had no further worries on this particular problem. The trustees were relieved of their stand-by duties and I have to thank them for being at hand and forever vigilant. Of course I miss Cynthia terribly and there are times when I can feel her presence in the home, and I admit to talking to her and then I pull myself together and say to myself 'well that was a nice little interlude'. Cynthia had such a quiet but somehow pleasantly domineering attitude which will never be swept away. I very sincerely hope that she and her Mum are enjoying each other's company and I hope you will not think I am becoming too sentimental. I now think I should end this story of an experience and proceed with some not to be forgotten business.

Prior to moving on to the penultimate chapter, I would like to comment generally on those who suffer from cerebral palsy in view of the fact that I have been personally involved and tried to prosecute cause and effect. I consider that I have an opinion to pass on to those similarly affected. It is only an opinion and not a decisive answer to this terrible affliction, I am not qualified to register other than this.

I have been prompted to emerge with certain comments following my viewing of a film on television named *My Left Foot*. I am sure many thousands of viewers will have devoted time to this brilliant exposition of first of all a young lad, and later a grown-up victim of cerebral palsy who had been taught and who discovered that he could carry out many functions and actions with his left foot. It was a very significant achievement and one worthy of showing. His behaviour towards the end of the film left something to be desired and I felt that perhaps he had been pushed too far, for he let himself and his supporters down, and I feel sure that he personally could not be blamed, having regard to the state of his unsettled brain together with the multitude of emotions he was unable to control. Perhaps here we might reflect carefully as carers in such cases.

This brings me to the point as to why I referred to the above film, and how Rene and I faced up to such a challenge. There came a period after our journeys across the country seeking help and advice, when my wife and I began to discuss the possibilities of educating Cynthia and also whether physiotherapy would help her to use her arms and legs. We decided to discuss the problems with our doctor − he was always ready to listen and help. He passed on some advice which I have never forgotten. The text of this statement was: "By all means try to carry out your plans, but I would warn you not to press the girl too far. She has a sweet nature which is worth holding on to, don't run the risk of destroying this or your own lives could become more difficult." Actually this turned out to be wise advice and Rene and I decided to carry on as we were going, to allow Cynthia to listen to as much radio as possible and eventually television. This paid off from the educative point of view and she became quite brilliant at memorising and also with her music appreciation.

However, I submit this to parents similarly affected, and ask them to draw some conclusions especially to my remarks concerning *My Left Foot*. In short, do not push you luck too far, it could have horrendous effects generally. We must not forget that the damage to the brain has occurred much earlier in life, and that damaged brain has to be succoured and not overtaxed or abused.

Chapter Twelve

This is the penultimate chapter and is to be one of dedication towards those who have helped Cynthia, her Mum and myself over this era of varied situations comprising concerns, pleasures and disappointments but with endeavour to always trying to bring about change with possible success. Unfortunately not always a winner but not lacking in the effort to try to succeed.

To two people whom I have not mentioned before and relating to our early days in Falmouth I must not forget Mr and Mrs Strongman, both now deceased but whom Cynthia became very attached to and they to her. They could not help her very much but the thought was there. She was able to give support to Mrs Strongman to no end when Mr Strongman died and this continued right up to Mrs Strongman's decease. It was a strange associationship but there was something born within Cynthia that she always wanted to be helpful and comforting to those she loved.

Also in such a similar case I consider I ought to mention the help and sincerity of two people who were very close to us in our adversity, if such it should be called. They are Marjorie and Geoff Hillier who lived close to us when we first lived in Falmouth and then later when we moved to Penryn. Geoff has now died but Marjorie still lives on in her birth county of Wiltshire. Herein we experienced a very good sample of Christianity as it should be practised.

I must now move on to those whom I have named *My Magnificent Seven*. The ladies and gentlemen who gave me absolute support from the day I returned to Falmouth with Cynthia and who have been a tower of strength to me both before and following Cynthia's decease. They are, and I proudly name:

> Mrs Jean Trevena
> Mr Walter Trevena
> Miss Heather Trevena
> Mrs Wendy Dean
> Mr Colin Dean
> Mrs Jan Mullett
> Mr Rob Mullett

They are all good friends together but please forgive me for emulating Jean, Walter and Heather Trevena for our associationship, love and caring for over thirty years. I feel sure the other four named persons would agree and not feel ensconsed. I have to specifically say that these good friends took Cynthia to their hearts, made arrangements to take her into their homes so that she was never left to herself, and she enjoyed it. She gained confidence by such treatment and they, the Magnificent Seven, knew exactly what sort of a world they were trying to create for her.

I have a special word to say about Steven Dean, son of Wendy and Colin. As a youngster of some twelve years old he came into this house and attached himself to Cynthia, I was quite surprised and they became great friends. Similarly there was no doubting the friendship coming from Gavin and Paul Mullett. They had all been educated obviously that not everyone was quite as lucky as they were. Incidentally, I was very elated and so was Cynthia because she never ever showed it but she knew when others were backing off. I am sorry to have to relate to such things but it is an absolutely noticeable fact of life.

I would be in error if I neglected to express my appreciation of first of all our Dr Oakens and his nursing staff from Modbury Health Centre in Devon, and Dr Davis and his nursing staff at Falmouth.

I would also be quite out of order not to refer to Cynthia's two other trustees, namely David and Nona Hillier. An especial word of thanks to them both.

I must refer to the help and assistance of some special friends relating to our years in Devonshire. Without them life would have become most difficult at times. Hereto I commend never forgetful thoughts to:

Linda and David Honey
Marjorie Hunt
Miss Hopper

All these friends came from the various hamlets, such as Hemerdon or Lutton, which were close to our main village of Sparkwell. They all were sorry we had to leave the district but they all knew it was for the best in the circumstances.

Chapter Thirteen

In bringing this rather unique, but very authentic, story to an end, I feel there are certain conclusions to be drawn, borne in mind and accentuated upon.

First of all, I personally, and earlier with my dear wife, never regretted the action we took to try and make ours a happy family. I would ask you to perhaps consider that we could have, in the early days, discarded our responsibilities to Cynthia and had her placed in care. I very much doubt if there are many parents who would take such action but it has been known to happen, of this I am sure. I think to further deliberate upon such decisions must be very private indeed.

However, arriving at 1987/88, it has now been established that children with cerebral palsy can be treated with some successful outcome at two clinics, one in Switzerland and another in Budapest, Hungary, which leads me to evoke "What about Britain?" Both the clinics referred to abroad are very expensive for ordinary people to manage, and one reads of a number of fund-raising ventures to provide the wherewithal for various unfortunate children to be privileged to attend such institutions. But some success has been definitely achieved and that is progress, of course.

Which leads me to remark what is wrong with Britain's

60

surgical teams? And here we are with supposedly the finest health service in the world. To a person like myself, and I have explained how we tried over the years, I ought to feel embittered — but I do not, I feel that every effort we made must have encouraged our medical profession to some sort of research. A lack of funds has perhaps allowed the Continent to overtake us. I must leave you and similar parents as myself to draw your own conclusions. It has recently been established that at least four British therapists are being trained at the Peto Institute in Budapest. There is hope yet!

It is obvious from a general point of view that our disabled establishment do not achieve sufficient support to assist them to overcome their problems. Great progress has been made to help this tragic society with such benefits as Attendance Allowance, Mobility Allowance and special units set up to assist immobile patients to walk etc. Now in the latter instance these units are severely underfunded. This cannot be right and our National Health Service is sadly lacking herein. I feel that we should pursue the progress made in the Continental countries, because for some reason, probably underfunding, we and our very proficient medical teams fail to make the equivalent progress necessary.

My last conclusion is so simple that it ought to be made law.

A lot of success has been achieved in the procurement of suitable access points for disabled persons in wheel-chairs but not one hundred per cent, there are still many buildings lacking in this facility. Also if you as parents are financially sound enough you can, as I have on three occasions, buy suitable vehicles for conversion to suit your personal needs in order to make life easy family-wise. Please bear in mind that I said if you are financially sound enough, and I would emphasise that a lot of parents and the unfortunate recipients of such crippling disadvantages are unable to take advantage without the help of Mobility Allowance, which does not cover the cost of everything nor does it cover the time lag to achieve some satisfactory result.

We are drawing conclusions and I would ask you to relate to my experience when I moved from Devon back to Cornwall — a move which had been planned to absolute detail so as not to upset the general routine of our patient, Cynthia. The only real devastation was the type of hoist supplied by the County Council for our use at home. Upon complaint, to be told that there was nothing they could do to supply a suitable hoist was really a very disappointing phenomena. I hesitate to further comment upon this, because I have already explained how we achieved our aim, but this occurrence is a fair example of what our unfortunate folk have to suffer. Why should this be? I ask and I deliver the foregoing statement, unless you can face up to it and fight like a demon, you will go under, and this sort of situation must stop. I have to ask you to consider that some parents can fight and some cannot and the patient, whoever he or she may be, may be fortunate or otherwise.

I have achieved as a result of my experience a feeling that we are an overlooked society. The whole associated conditions in which we try to survive should be thoroughly investigated and whilst I survive I shall be fighting to be successful in this juncture. Just two final comments. Firstly, is it really necessary that people with such problems should always be at war with bureaucracy? I think not, because most of us are very genuine folk but the victims of circumstances beyond our control. Please also just reflect upon the two instances which I have described when Cynthia had to be taken into hospital. Do you not feel that there is a sad lack of detail and attention in such cases? What can be done about it?

Secondly, it seems nowadays that steep financial compensations can be achieved, perhaps up to one million pounds, if it can be proved that the cerebral palsy is caused by some medical neglect or misadventure at birth. So by the processes of pre-birth conditions and now present-day progress in medical science, something has been achieved. Money however, will never be a substitute for a really healthy human being, but it does help a lot to provide comforts and assistance to parents who have a lifetime of awareness and attachment to look forward to. Therefore one has to assume some ratification for mistakes.

I think I can safely say to present-day unfortunate parents, things could be much worse for you. I know, but for a safe and qualified job, I would have been declared bankrupt. Instead I feel very proud, as I know my late wife was, to have overcome the unfortunate handicap we had to face, to the best of our ability.

If I can achieve publication of this book, which I sincerely hope will be the case, I will personally be responsible for a copy to be placed in the most appropriate places. It is my sincere wish to achieve more help and consideration for this overlooked section of society.

Appendix

There is a small but important area which ought to be referred to, but I did not feel it was really part of the intended import of the book in particular. Now this concerns structural details within the confines of where one might live. If in a house, one should make the effort to change to a bungalow. All mums and dads, other members of the family and the patient himself most importantly, will find life a whole lot easier especially when using wheel-chairs, maybe commodes and especially the hoist lifter.

I am able to say that I was lucky, working in the construction trade, and so preparatory alterations came easier to me than most. Therefore I would like to add the following structural ideas to give families some idea of how to cope – any good builder should be able to advise accordingly.

The general idea must be to make for more room. All internal doors should be not less than 2ft 9" wide, and all passageways not less than 4ft wide. When designing a new property, all this should be easy to deal with. When altering an existing property life becomes more difficult, so take the advice of a reputable builder or building surveyor.

The next stage is very important as it concerns the patient's bedroom and bathroom, and both should be in close proximity to the other. Efforts should be made to site the bed head on to a wall and in a central position so that access is available to both sides of the bed. This, for obvious reasons, is to assist and make two persons available for any lifting or change of position of the patient. Transfer of the patient to the bathroom may of course be by the hoist lifter. Again plenty of room is needed and a bathroom of not less than 10ft square. The bath should be fixed in the centre of one wall with its length protruding into the room. Again this position allows access to both sides of the patient whilst bathing is carried out. Patience and dedication usually finds ways round difficult situations which usually crop up, and a smile from the patient makes everything worthwhile.

Access to front, back and any garden doors should allow for concrete ramps to assist handling of wheel-chairs. Grants are available from local councils to assist financially with structural alterations.

Below is a sketch plan illustrating the points I have made. Any further help or advice — I shall be an ever open door!

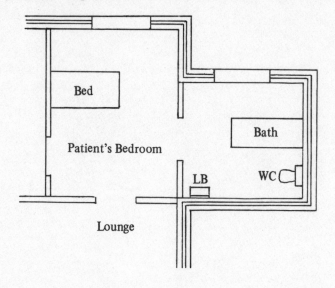